Living well
Beyond
Kidney Disease

Subtitle:

Strategies for a Full Life

Dr. Sharon C. Stallworth

Table of content

Introduction

- Personal story or case study illustrating the possibility of living well beyond kidney disease.
- The Value of a positive mindset and determination when dealing with kidney disease.
- brief overview of what you can expect from the pages that follow

Certainly, the following personal experience can demonstrate the possibility of surviving kidney disease for a very long time:

Meet Halima Abdussalam, a wonderful woman whose life took a sudden turn when she was given the news that she had kidney illness in her early 20s. Her entire universe appeared to collapse at that precise instant. She had a difficult journey ahead of her, one that was paved with doctor's appointments, treatments, and doubt about her future.

Halima had challenges during her battle with kidney disease. The effects of having a chronic illness on her included exhaustion, dietary restrictions, and mental stress. Halima stands out, though, for her strong resolve to not allow kidney disease dictate how she lives.

She started looking into her illness Halima started to see new possibilities as she dove into her condition's studies and connected with other patients and support organizations. She learned that she could live a happy life despite her condition. Halima accepted her course of treatment, collaborated extensively with her medical staff, and changed her lifestyle significantly.

Halima is now thriving rather than merely getting by. She is a champion for raising awareness of kidney disease, a motivator for those suffering comparable difficulties, and a brilliant example of what is possible when you don't allow a condition to define you.

This book contains numerous stories, like Halima's, that demonstrate the enormous possibility for a full and fulfilling life despite renal disease. Continue reading to learn how to build a life that goes well beyond renal disease, use your own inner resources and strength, just like Halima did.

The Value of a Positive Mindset and Determination When Dealing with Kidney diseases

In the face of a kidney disease diagnosis, it's natural to experience a whirlwind of emotions – fear, uncertainty, and even a sense of loss. The journey ahead may appear daunting, filled with medical appointments, treatments, and lifestyle adjustments. However, amidst these challenges, one of the most potent tools at your disposal is your mindset.

Having a positive mindset, coupled with unwavering determination, can be a beacon of hope during your kidney disease journey. Here's why it matters:

1. Enhancing Resilience: Having a positive outlook does not mean you should downplay your struggles. Instead, the focus should be on strengthening one's ability to face obstacles head-on. You're more likely to succeed when you tackle kidney disease with a positive outlook.

2. Stress Reduction: Stress can have an adverse effect on your general wellbeing and increase kidney disease symptoms. Keeping a good attitude can assist lower stress levels, which can improve health outcomes. It's a good cycle: reduced stress leads to improved health,

which promotes happier attitudes.

3. Improving Quality of Life:Your attitude can significantly influence your quality of life. A positive mindset can make the journey more enjoyable and fulfilling. It can help you find joy in everyday experiences, maintain social connections, and pursue your passions.

4. Enhancing Treatment Adherence:Staying motivated and determined can improve your adherence to treatment plans, including medications, dietary restrictions, and lifestyle changes. When you believe in the importance of your treatment and its potential benefits, you're more likely to follow it consistently.

5. Empowering Self-Advocacy:A positive mindset can empower you to take an active role in your healthcare journey.

You'll be more inclined to ask questions, seek second opinions, and advocate for your needs. This sense of empowerment can lead to better communication with your healthcare team and more personalized care.

6. Inspiring Others: Your positive mindset can inspire those around you, including family, friends, and fellow kidney disease patients. By embodying resilience and determination, you become a source of hope and motivation for others facing similar challenges.

7. Fostering Hope: Kidney disease may alter your life, but it doesn't have to define it. A positive mindset fosters hope for a better future, one where you continue to pursue your dreams, set goals, and find fulfillment despite the condition.

Though there may be challenging days along the way, keep in mind that there will also be days that are full of optimism, advancement, and successes as you navigate your kidney disease journey. Those fleeting moments of hope might become a reality thanks to the power of your attitude. Utilize the strength of optimism and steadfast resolve as you travel the road to a life free from renal disease.

Brief Summary of What to Expect from the Pages that Follow

With this book, "Living Well Beyond Kidney Disease – Strategies for a Full Life," we set out to investigate kidney disease in great detail. Our mission is to give you a road map, direction, and inspiration so that you can not only survive with renal disease but also thrive in spite of it.

What follows is a brief summary of what to expect from the pages that follow:

1. Understanding Kidney Disease: Let's start by dispelling some myths about kidneys and their functions. You'll learn more about kidney disease,

including its causes and various kinds. We'll provide you the information you need to completely understand your condition.

2. Navigating the Diagnosis: We'll explore the psychological effects of being told you have kidney illness and provide resources to assist you in coping. On this voyage, you'll come to realize that you're not alone.

3. Treatment Options: You'll investigate a range of treatment options, including prescription drugs, dialysis, and transplantation. We'll stress the value of individualized treatment programs created specifically for your individual requirements.

4. Lifestyle and Diet for Kidney Health: Understand how lifestyle and nutritional decisions can be crucial in controlling renal disease. On nutrition, physical

activity, and general wellbeing, we'll offer helpful advice.

5. Coping with Challenges: Recognize how to deal with potential symptoms, discomfort, and emotional obstacles. The real-life experiences of those who have overcome these obstacles will serve as inspiration.

6. Empowering Your Mindset: Understand the enormous power of having a positive outlook. We'll go over ways to develop and accomplish goals, stay motivated, and reach your maximum potential.

7. Building a Support System: Develop a solid support system with your friends, family, medical professionals, and support groups. You can navigate these crucial connections with the use of effective communication techniques.

8. Advocacy and Awareness:Learn how you can participate in

campaigns to raise awareness of renal illness. You'll learn about those who have significantly impacted this field.

9. Planning for the Future: Consider your renal disease prognosis over the long run. We'll talk about financial planning and offer advice on how to develop and accomplish objectives for your life besides kidney disease.)

Chapter 1: Understanding Kidney Disease

Kidneys and their Functions

The kidneys are essential organs in the human body that are placed on either side of the spine, just below the ribcage, and are roughly the size of a fist. They play an important role in general health by fulfilling numerous key functions:

1. Filtration: The kidneys' principal role is to filter and eliminate waste products, excessive salts, and excessive fluids from the bloodstream. These waste materials are then expelled in the form of urine.

2. Blood Pressure Control: Kidneys help regulate blood pressure by managing the volume of blood as well as the amount of sodium and water in the body. They produce renin, a hormone that is important in blood pressure regulation.

3. Electrolyte Balance: Kidneys keep electrolytes like sodium, potassium, and calcium in balance in the body, which is essential for nerve and muscle function.

4. Acid-Base Balance: They aid in the maintenance of the body's pH by excreting hydrogen ions and reabsorbing bicarbonate ions.

5. Erythropoiesis Control: The kidneys manufacture and release erythropoietin, a hormone that drives red blood cell formation in the bone marrow.

6. Excretion of Toxins: The kidneys filter and eliminate

numerous toxins and medications from the bloodstream.

7. Water Balance: They regulate the amount of water discharged in urine, which aids in the prevention of dehydration and excessive fluid retention.

Overall, the kidneys are necessary for the body to maintain a stable internal environment, and their optimal operation is critical for optimum health.

Explanation of what kidney disease is, it's causes and its types

Kidney Disease

Kidney Disease, also known as renal disease, is a disorder in which the kidneys are damaged and can not filter blood rightly, causing waste accoutrements and fluids to accumulate in the body. This can beget a variety of health issues. Chronic kidney disease (CKD), acute kidney injury(AKI), and numerous beginning causes similar as diabetes, high blood pressure, infections, and others are all exemplifications of kidney Disease. Treatment styles differ depending on the disease kind and stage. To avoid difficulties, early detection and care are essential.

Causes of kidney Disease

Kidney disease can have various causes, and it's essential to identify and address the underlying factor to manage or prevent further kidney damage. Here are some common causes of kidney disease:
1. Diabetes:Uncontrolled high blood sugar levels over time can damage the small blood vessels in the kidneys, leading to diabetic kidney disease (nephropathy).
2.Hypertension (High Blood Pressure): Persistent high blood pressure can strain the blood vessels in the kidneys, impairing their ability to filter waste and fluids effectively.
3. Glomerulonephritis:This is an inflammation of the glomeruli, which are the small filtering units in the kidneys. It can be caused by infections, immune system disorders, or other conditions.

4. Polycystic Kidney Disease (PKD):A genetic disorder characterized by the growth of fluid-filled cysts in the kidneys, which can lead to kidney damage over time.

5. Autoimmune Diseases: Conditions like lupus and vasculitis can affect the kidneys by causing inflammation and damage to the filtering structures.

6. Kidney Stones:Hard deposits of minerals and salts can form in the kidneys, blocking urine flow and potentially causing damage.

7. Urinary Tract Obstruction:Blockages in the urinary tract, such as due to tumors, kidney stones, or an enlarged prostate, can prevent proper urine flow and harm the kidneys.

8. Infections:Severe infections, especially those affecting the urinary tract or causing sepsis, can lead to kidney damage.

9. Medications and Toxins:Certain medications, such as non-steroidal anti-inflammatory drugs (NSAIDs), antibiotics, and contrast dyes used in imaging, can be

nephrotoxic (toxic to the kidneys).

10. Dehydration: Insufficient fluid intake or conditions causing excessive fluid loss, like vomiting, diarrhea, or heatstroke, can strain the kidneys and lead to injury.

11. Hereditary Factors: Some kidney diseases have a genetic component, meaning they run in families. Examples include Alport syndrome and some forms of PKD.

12. Aging:As people age, kidney function naturally declines. This is called age-related kidney degeneration.

13. Heart Disease: Heart conditions that affect blood flow can indirectly harm the kidneys.

14. Smoking and Substance Abuse:These can contribute to kidney damage over time.

15. Obesity:Excess body weight and fat can increase the risk of developing kidney disease.

It's important to note that early detection and management of underlying conditions, lifestyle modifications (e.g., maintaining a healthy diet and regular exercise), and avoiding nephrotoxic substances can help prevent or slow the progression of kidney disease. Regular check-ups and monitoring kidney function are crucial for individuals at risk or with existing kidney problems.

Types of kidney Disease

Certainly, there are several types and causes of kidney disease. Here are some of common ones:

1. Chronic Kidney Disease (CKD): A long-term condition where the kidneys gradually lose their function over time. It is often caused by conditions like diabetes, high blood pressure, or other chronic diseases.

2. Acute Kidney Injury (AKI): Sudden and temporary loss of kidney function, often due to severe infections, dehydration, medications, or trauma.

3. Polycystic Kidney Disease (PKD): A genetic disorder characterized by the growth of numerous cysts in the kidneys, which can impair their function.

4. Glomerulonephritis: Inflammation of the glomeruli, the tiny filtering units in the kidneys, often resulting from

immune system disorders or infections.

5. Diabetic Nephropathy: Kidney damage caused by diabetes, primarily due to long-term high blood sugar levels.

6. Hypertensive Nephropathy: Kidney damage resulting from prolonged high blood pressure, which can impair the kidneys' ability to filter blood effectively.

7. Kidney Stones: Hard deposits of minerals and salts that can form in the kidneys and cause pain when they pass through the urinary tract.

8. Inherited Kidney Diseases: Various genetic conditions, such as Alport syndrome and Fabry disease, can lead to kidney dysfunction.

9. Interstitial Nephritis: Inflammation of the kidney's tubules and surrounding tissue, often caused by medications or infections.

10. Obstructive Uropathy: Blockage of the urinary tract, which can lead to kidney damage. Causes may include kidney stones, tumors, or congenital abnormalities.

11.Nephrotic Syndrome: A group of symptoms indicating kidney damage, including proteinuria (excess protein in urine), edema (swelling), and high cholesterol.

12. Renal Artery Stenosis: Narrowing of the arteries that supply blood to the kidneys, typically due to atherosclerosis, which can lead to hypertension and kidney problems.

These are just some of the many types and causes of kidney disease, each requiring different approaches to diagnosis and treatment. It's essential to consult a healthcare professional for proper evaluation and management if you suspect kidney issues.

Chronic Kidney Disease (CKD)

- **Definition**: CKD is a long-term, progressive condition in which the kidneys gradually lose their ability to function properly over an extended period. It's often characterized by the slow and irreversible decline in kidney function.

- **Stages**: CKD is typically categorized into stages based on the estimated Glomerular Filtration Rate (eGFR), which measures how effectively the kidneys filter waste from the blood. The stages are as follows:

1. Stage 1: eGFR > 90 mL/min/1.73 m² - Kidney damage with normal or high filtration rate.
2. Stage 2: eGFR 60-89 mL/min/1.73 m² - Mildly reduced kidney function.
3. Stage 3: eGFR 30-59 mL/min/1.73 m² - Moderately reduced kidney function.
4. Stage 4: eGFR 15-29 mL/min/1.73 m² - Severely reduced kidney function.
5. Stage 5 (End-Stage Renal Disease or ESRD):
 eGFR < 15 mL/min/1.73 m² - Kidney failure requiring dialysis or transplantation for survival.

- **Causes**: CKD can result from various underlying conditions, including:

- Diabetes: High blood sugar levels can harm the kidney's tiny blood vessels.

- Hypertension: Prolonged high blood pressure can harm the kidney's filtering units (glomeruli).

- Glomerulonephritis: Inflammation of the glomeruli, often due to immune system disorders or infections.

- Polycystic Kidney Disease (PKD): A genetic disorder leading to the growth of cysts in the kidneys.

- Other conditions: Kidney stones, urinary tract obstructions, autoimmune diseases, and more.

- **Symptoms**: CKD may be asymptomatic in its early stages. As it progresses, common symptoms and complications can include:

- Fatigue
- Swelling (edema)
- Increased or decreased urine output
- High blood pressure
- Anemia
- Bone and mineral disorders
- Electrolyte imbalances
- Cardiovascular issues
- Neuropathy
- Itchy skin
- Nausea and vomiting

- **Diagnosis**: CKD is typically diagnosed through blood tests measuring serum creatinine levels, urine tests to assess proteinuria or hematuria, and calculating eGFR. Imaging studies like ultrasounds or CT scans may also be used to identify structural abnormalities.
- **Treatment**: Management of CKD involves:

1. Addressing the underlying cause (e.g., controlling blood sugar or blood pressure).
2. Medications to manage symptoms and complications (e.g. antihypertensives, erythropoietin for anemia).
3. Lifestyle changes (e.g. dietary modifications, exercise, smoking cessation).
4. Dialysis in advanced stages or kidney transplantation for ESRD.

- **Prognosis**: CKD progression can vary widely, and early detection and management are crucial for slowing its advancement. Some individuals may remain stable in the early stages for many years, while others may progress more rapidly. ESRD requires ongoing dialysis or transplantation for survival.

NB: Regular monitoring and collaboration with healthcare providers are essential for individuals with CKD to optimize their quality of life and manage the condition effectively.

Acute Kidney Injury (AKI)

- **Definition**: Acute Kidney Injury, formerly known as acute renal failure, is a sudden and often reversible loss of kidney function, occurring over a short period of time, typically within hours to a few days.
- **Causes**

1. Dehydration: One of the most common causes is severe dehydration, often due to insufficient fluid intake or excessive fluid loss from

conditions like vomiting, diarrhea, or excessive sweating.

2. Medications: Certain medications, especially those that can be toxic to the kidneys, such as non-steroidal anti-inflammatory drugs (NSAIDs), some antibiotics, and contrast agents used in imaging procedures, can trigger AKI.

3. Infections: Severe infections, like sepsis, can lead to AKI due to the release of toxins into the bloodstream.

4. Trauma: Physical injuries, surgery, or trauma that directly affects the kidneys or the blood flow to the kidneys can result in AKI.

5. Kidney Obstruction: Conditions that obstruct the urinary tract, such as kidney stones or tumors, can disrupt normal urine flow and cause AKI.

6. Autoimmune Diseases: Autoimmune conditions like lupus or vasculitis can damage the kidneys' filtering units, leading to AKI.

7. Hemodynamic Changes: Abrupt changes in blood pressure, including extremely

low blood pressure (hypotension) or extremely high blood pressure (hypertension), can affect kidney function.

- **Symptoms**:

AKI may present with symptoms like decreased urine output, swelling (edema), fatigue, confusion, nausea, and shortness of breath. However, these symptoms can vary depending on the underlying cause and severity of the injury.

- **Diagnosis**:

Diagnosis involves evaluating a patient's medical history, conducting physical exams, and running various tests, including blood tests to assess kidney function (e.g., creatinine and blood urea nitrogen levels), urine tests, and imaging studies like ultrasounds or CT scans.

- **Stages**:

AKI is typically classified into three stages based on the severity of kidney dysfunction: Stage 1 (mild), Stage 2 (moderate), and Stage 3 (severe). The staging helps guide treatment decisions.

- **Treatment**:

Management of AKI often depends on the underlying cause.

Treatment may include addressing the cause (e.g., treating an infection), fluid and electrolyte balance management, avoiding nephrotoxic medications, and providing supportive care like dialysis when necessary to help filter the blood while the kidneys recover.

- **Prognosis**:

AKI can be reversible, especially when identified and treated promptly. However, severe cases can lead to chronic kidney disease (CKD) if not managed appropriately. The prognosis varies based on the cause, the patient's overall health, and the timeliness of intervention.

Early recognition and treatment of the underlying cause are crucial in improving outcomes for individuals with AKI. Monitoring kidney function and managing risk factors are essential to prevent recurrence.

The Importance of Early Detection and Diagnosis

The Value of Early Detection and Diagnosis:

When it comes to kidney disease, timing is crucial. It's like spotting a tiny fracture in a dam before it develops into a major breach. Because of this, the significance of early detection and diagnosis reverberates throughout our trip.

1. A Quiet Opponent

Early kidney disease is a master of disguising itself. It is a silent enemy that frequently advances without causing worry through observable signs. This covert phase might give us a false feeling of security, leading us to think everything is well when the disease is actually subtly progressing.

2. The Opportunity Window

A critical window of opportunity is opened by early detection. It's the time when we can step in and start using medications and altering our lifestyles to stop kidney disease before it even starts. This window gets smaller and our options to maintain renal function grow more limited the later we detect the disease.

3. Lightening the Load

Kidney illness can be physically and psychologically taxing, especially in its severe stages.

Early detection may help us lessen the severity of its symptoms, complications, and emotional toll on our life.

4. Providing Options

Early diagnosis gives us freedom of choice. It enables us to collaborate directly with medical professionals to create a customized treatment plan catered to our particular set of circumstances. We can investigate many treatment alternatives, actively participate in our care, and make well-informed decisions regarding our health.

5. Positivity and Hope

Detection that occurs early offers hope. It provides us with grounds for hope for the future. It serves as a reminder that we have the ability to take control of our health, make healthy lifestyle adjustments, and steer clear of kidney disease's limitations.

We will look at strategies to protect your health and look for early detection in the chapters that follow. We'll talk about the value of routine exams, comprehending risk factors, and picking up on minor symptoms that could otherwise go unreported. Beginning with the sobering realization that early identification can be a game-changer, giving us the chance to sculpt a happier and healthier future, is where our journey toward living well beyond kidney disease begins.

Common misconceptions and fears about kidney disease

<u>Misconceptions</u>:

1. Only Older People Get Kidney Disease: Kidney disease can affect people of all ages, including children and young adults. It's not solely an age-related condition.

2. Kidney Disease is Always Symptomatic: Early stages of kidney disease may not exhibit noticeable symptoms. Regular check-ups and blood tests are essential for early detection.

3. Kidney Disease Only Happens to Unhealthy People: While certain

lifestyle factors can increase the risk, kidney disease can also affect individuals with no history of poor health.

4. Dialysis Cures Kidney Disease: Dialysis is a treatment that helps manage kidney failure but doesn't cure the underlying condition. Kidney transplants are sometimes necessary for a cure.

5. Kidney Disease is Always Inherited: Many cases of kidney disease are not hereditary; they result from other factors like diabetes or hypertension.

6. Kidney Disease is Rare: Kidney disease is more common than people realize, with millions of individuals affected worldwide.

<u>Fears</u>:

1. Fear of Dialysis: Many people with kidney disease fear undergoing dialysis, which can be a life-saving treatment but requires regular sessions and lifestyle adjustments.

2. Fear of Transplant: While kidney transplantation can offer a cure, there's often fear associated with the surgery, finding a compatible donor, and potential complications.

3. Fear of Lifestyle Changes: Managing kidney disease often involves significant lifestyle changes, such as dietary restrictions and medication regimens, which can be overwhelming.

4. Fear of Progression: Patients may fear that their kidney disease will worsen over time, leading to more complications and a reduced quality of life.

5. Fear of Financial Burden: The costs associated with kidney disease treatment, including medications, dialysis, and transplantation, can be a source of anxiety for patients and their families.

6. Fear of Dependency: Kidney disease can sometimes lead to a sense of dependency on medical

treatments and healthcare providers, which can be emotionally challenging.

7. Fear of Social Stigma: Some individuals fear social isolation or discrimination due to their kidney disease, especially if they require dialysis or transplantation.

- In Chapter 1, we embarked on a journey into the world of kidney disease, a journey not of fear, but of understanding, empowerment, and hope. We have peeled back the layers, demystifying this condition that might have seemed daunting at first. As we conclude this chapter, let's reflect on the valuable insights we've gained:

1. Knowledge as a Beacon of Hope
2. Challenges and opportunities
3. A community of support
4. A road head.

So, as we close this chapter, do so with a heart filled with understanding, a mind ignited

with knowledge, and a spirit infused with hope. The journey continues, and together, we shall explore every facet of living well beyond kidney disease.

Chapter 2: Navigating the Diagnosis

How to cope with the emotional impact of a kidney disease diagnosis

Coping with the Emotional Impact of a Kidney Disease Diagnosis.
Receiving a kidney disease diagnosis can be a life-altering moment, one that reverberates with a mix of emotions—fear, confusion, anger, and uncertainty. It's natural to feel overwhelmed, but it's also crucial to recognize that your emotional well-being is an integral part of your journey toward living well beyond kidney disease. In this chapter, we'll explore not only the emotional challenges that

may arise but also practical strategies to cope and thrive.

Understanding the Emotional Rollercoaster

First and foremost, let's acknowledge that your emotional responses are valid. From the initial shock of the diagnosis to the ongoing adjustments required, kidney disease often triggers a roller coaster of feelings. You're not alone in experiencing these emotions, and it's essential to give yourself permission to feel and express them.

The Power of Self-Compassion

Amidst the emotional turmoil, self-compassion becomes your greatest ally. We'll delve into the art of treating yourself with the same kindness and understanding that you would offer a dear friend facing a similar challenge. Self-compassion can help you navigate the emotional labyrinth with greater resilience.

Building a Support System

One of the most powerful resources for coping emotionally is the support of loved ones. We'll discuss how to open up to friends and family about your feelings and needs, fostering a network of understanding and empathy. Additionally, we'll explore the role of professional support, from therapists to support groups, in providing you with the tools to process and manage your emotions effectively.

Mindfulness and Emotional Resilience

The practice of mindfulness can be a game-changer in coping with the emotional impact of kidney disease. We'll introduce you to mindfulness techniques that can help you stay grounded in the present moment, manage stress, and cultivate emotional resilience.

Setting Realistic Goals and Expectations

Kidney disease may necessitate adjustments in your life, but it doesn't diminish your capacity for meaningful achievements and personal growth. We'll explore the process of setting realistic goals and expectations, allowing you to focus on what truly matters and find purpose in your journey.

Stories of Triumph

Throughout this chapter, you'll find inspiring stories of individuals who have not only coped with the emotional challenges of kidney disease but have also emerged stronger, more resilient, and with a deeper appreciation for life. Their journeys will remind you that, even in the midst of emotional turbulence, there is hope and the potential for transformation.
In this point, we embark on a voyage through the seas of emotion, charting a course toward emotional well-being and resilience. Remember, while kidney disease may introduce complexity into your life, it also offers an opportunity to discover your inner strength and the power to shape your emotional landscape.

Resources for finding support and understanding from healthcare professionals and support groups.

Charting a Course Through Compassionate Care

In this section, we navigate the complex landscape of kidney disease with the aim of empowering you with the resources and support necessary for your journey. Kidney disease, like any medical condition, can be a labyrinthine path, often fraught with uncertainty. It's during these moments that a guiding hand and empathetic voices can make all the difference.

The Compassionate Care Network:
Discover the vital role healthcare professionals play in your journey. From nephrologists to dietitians and nurses, you'll learn how to build a trusted team of experts who are not just well-versed in kidney disease but also dedicated to providing compassionate care.

Unveiling the Power of Knowledge:
- How to find the right healthcare professionals who understand your unique needs.
- Tips for effective communication with your medical team.

- The importance of being an informed patient and advocate for your own care.

The Strength of Community

Beyond the clinical realm, support groups and communities are pillars of strength for individuals facing kidney disease. This section unveils the power of shared experiences and the profound understanding that comes from connecting with others who are on a similar path.

Navigating the Support Group Landscape:

- Where to find kidney disease support groups, both online and in your local community.
- How to participate in and benefit from these groups.
- Heartfelt stories of individuals whose lives have been transformed through support and solidarity.

Additional Resources at Your Fingertips

We've curated a wealth of additional resources to further guide you on your quest for support and understanding. From reputable websites to organizations dedicated to kidney health, you'll have a comprehensive toolkit to aid you on your journey.

An Abundance of Knowledge Awaits:

- A directory of trusted online resources and organizations specializing in kidney health.

- Personal anecdotes from individuals who have found hope and help through these resources.

- Tips for effectively navigating the wealth of information available to you.

- Chapter 2 is your roadmap to not only understanding the intricacies of kidney disease but also to finding the compassionate care and support you deserve. As you continue your journey, remember that you are never alone. There is a network of professionals and a community of kindred spirits ready to walk alongside you, offering support and understanding every step of the way.

Chapter 3: Treatment Options

Overview of various treatment options, including medications, dialysis, and transplantation.

In the labyrinth of kidney disease, the path to wellness is illuminated by a spectrum of treatment possibilities. This Chapter is your compass, guiding you through this intricate terrain, where choices take shape, and hope is rekindled. Here, we embark on a journey to explore the diverse treatment options at your disposal, each offering a unique pathway toward kidney health.

Unveiling the Mosaic of Treatments

Imagine standing before a grand mosaic, its pieces representing the various treatments available for kidney disease. As we step closer, these pieces come into focus, each revealing its distinct role in your journey. Together, we'll understand the artistry behind treatments, including:

1. **Medications**: Delve into the world of pharmaceuticals designed to manage kidney disease. Discover how medications can alleviate symptoms, slow disease progression, and enhance your overall well-being. Gain insights into medication management, potential side effects, and the importance of medication adherence.

2. **Dialysis**: Dialysis artificially removes waste products and extra fluid from your blood when your kidneys can no longer do this. In hemodialysis, a machine filters waste and excess fluids from your blood. In peritoneal dialysis, a thin tube fitted into your tummy fills your abdominal depression with a dialysis result that absorbs waste and excess fluids. After a time, the dialysis result drains from your body, carrying the waste with it. Hemodialysis is more than a medical procedure; it's a bridge to a life well-lived despite kidney disease. As you journey

through this chapter, you'll be
equipped with the knowledge
and insights needed to make
informed decisions about
hemodialysis and to embark on a
path of empowerment and hope.
We'll navigate the intricate web
of dialysis, a lifeline for many
living with kidney disease.
Uncover the different types of
dialysis, their processes, and
what to expect during dialysis
sessions. Learn how dialysis can
empower you to lead a fulfilling
life while managing your
condition.

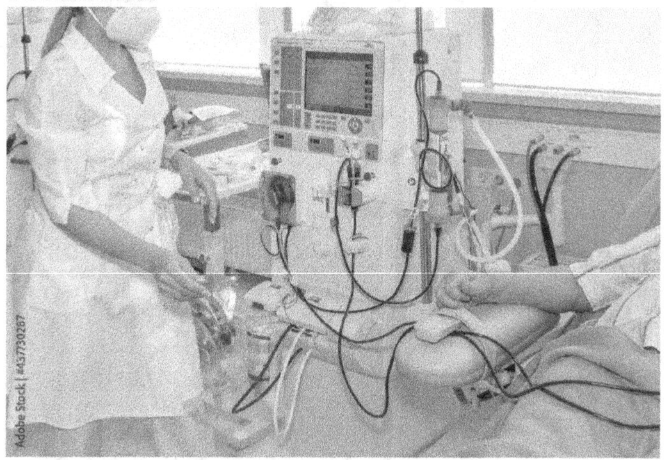

3. **Transplantation**: A kidney
transplant involves surgically
placing a healthy kidney from a
donor into your body.
Transplanted kidneys can come
from departed or living donors.
After a transplant, you will need

to take medications for the rest of your life to keep your body from rejecting the new organ. You do not need to be on dialysis to have a kidney transplant.

 A beacon of hope for many, kidney transplantation offers a chance at renewed vitality. We'll unravel the complexities of transplantation, from the evaluation process to the intricacies of finding a suitable donor. Explore the transformative impact of a successful kidney transplant on your life.

NB: For some who choose not to have dialysis or a kidney transplant, a third option is to treat your kidney failure with conservative measures.

Conservative measures probably will include symptom operation, advance care planning and care to keep you comfortable(palliative care)

Balancing the Scales of Choice

As we explore these treatment options, you'll gain a deeper understanding of the role they play in your unique journey. This chapter isn't about prescribing a singular path but empowering you with knowledge. It's about finding the treatment or combination of treatments that align with your goals, values, and aspirations.

Your Journey, Your Choices
Every person's journey through kidney disease is as unique as a fingerprint, and the treatment options you explore should reflect that individuality. This Chapter is your trusted guide as you consider the mosaic of treatments before you. It's about understanding, exploring, and ultimately, making choices that resonate with your vision for a life well-lived, beyond the confines of kidney disease.

some general advice for kidney patients regarding their treatment:
1. **Consult with a Nephrologist:** The first and most crucial step is to consult with a nephrologist, a kidney specialist. They will assess your condition, conduct necessary tests, and recommend the most appropriate treatment plan for you.
2. **Follow Medical Recommendations:** It's

essential to follow your
nephrologist's recommendations
diligently. This may include
taking prescribed medications,
undergoing regular tests, and
following dietary and lifestyle
guidelines.
3. **Stay Informed:** Educate
yourself about your kidney
condition. Understanding the
nature of your illness, available
treatments, and potential
complications can help you make
informed decisions and actively
participate in your care.
4. **Manage Your Diet:**
Kidney patients often require
specific dietary restrictions to
manage their condition. Follow
your healthcare provider's advice
regarding sodium, potassium,
phosphorus, and protein intake.
A registered dietitian can help
you create a personalized meal
plan.
5. **Stay Hydrated:** Adequate
hydration is crucial for kidney
health. However, the amount of
fluid you can consume may be
restricted, depending on your
condition. Work with your
healthcare team to determine the
right fluid intake for you.

6. **Regular Exercise:**
Consult with your healthcare
provider about an exercise plan
tailored to your condition.
Physical activity can help
improve overall health, manage
weight, and reduce the risk of
complications.
7. **Monitor Blood Pressure:**
High blood pressure is a common
issue for kidney patients.
Monitor your blood pressure
regularly, and take prescribed
medications to control it.
Lifestyle changes, such as
reducing salt intake and stress
management, can also help.
8. **Medication Management:**
Take your prescribed
medications as directed by your
healthcare provider. Don't skip
doses or make changes without
consulting them. Report any side
effects or concerns promptly.
9. **Quit Smoking and Limit
Alcohol:** Smoking and
excessive alcohol consumption
can worsen kidney problems. If
you smoke, seek support to quit,
and limit alcohol intake as
advised by your healthcare team.
10. **Mental Health:** Living
with a chronic illness can be

emotionally challenging. Don't hesitate to seek support from a therapist or counselor if you're struggling with anxiety, depression, or stress.

11. **Regular Follow-Up:** Attend all scheduled follow-up appointments with your nephrologist and other specialists involved in your care. Regular check-ups help monitor your progress and make necessary adjustments to your treatment plan.

12. **Engage in Support Groups:** Joining kidney disease support groups or online communities can provide valuable emotional support and a platform to exchange experiences and advice with others facing similar challenges.

Remember that kidney disease management is highly individualized. Your treatment plan may differ from others, depending on your specific condition and needs. Always consult with your healthcare provider for personalized guidance and adjustments to your treatment.

So, let's step closer to that mosaic together, unveiling the options that hold the potential to shape your path toward kidney health and a fulfilling future.

The role of healthcare providers in developing a personalized treatment plan.

The Role of Healthcare Providers in Personalized Treatment Plan are:

1. **Assessment and Diagnosis:** Healthcare providers begin by conducting a thorough assessment to diagnose the type and stage of kidney disease. They consider factors like kidney function, underlying causes, and any related health conditions.

2. **Individualized Evaluation:** Based on the assessment, healthcare providers tailor their approach to each patient. They take into account the patient's age, overall health, lifestyle, and preferences.

3. **Medication Management:** Healthcare providers prescribe medications to manage kidney

disease symptoms and slow its progression. The choice of medication and dosage is personalized to the patient's specific needs and any concurrent health issues.

4. **Dietary Guidance:** Diet plays a significant role in kidney health. Healthcare providers, often working with registered dietitians, create customized dietary plans that consider the patient's nutritional requirements, dietary restrictions, and stage of kidney disease.

5. **Fluid Management:** Kidney patients may need to monitor and restrict fluid intake. Healthcare providers provide guidance on the appropriate amount of fluids to consume based on individual circumstances.

6. **Blood Pressure Control:** Many kidney patients also have hypertension. Healthcare providers prescribe and adjust medications to maintain healthy blood pressure levels, reducing the strain on the kidneys.

7. **Treatment Decision-Making:** For advanced kidney disease, healthcare providers

discuss treatment options such as hemodialysis, peritoneal dialysis, or kidney transplantation. They help patients and their families make informed decisions aligned with their values and preferences.

8. **Regular Monitoring:** Healthcare providers schedule regular follow-up appointments to monitor kidney function and adjust treatment plans as needed. They may use lab tests, imaging, and other diagnostic tools to track progress.

9. **Pain and Symptom Management:** Kidney disease can cause discomfort and various symptoms. Healthcare providers address these symptoms, providing pain relief and improving the patient's overall quality of life.

10. **Emotional Support:** Dealing with chronic illness can be emotionally challenging. Healthcare providers offer emotional support and may refer patients to mental health professionals when needed.

11. **Patient Education:** One of the crucial roles of healthcare providers is to educate patients about their condition, treatment

options, and self-care. They empower patients with knowledge to actively participate in their care.

12. **Coordination of Care:** Healthcare providers often work in multidisciplinary teams, collaborating with nephrologists, nurses, dietitians, social workers, and other specialists to ensure holistic care for kidney patients.

13. **Advocacy:** Healthcare providers advocate for their patients, helping them access necessary services, navigate insurance and financial matters, and connect with support groups or community resources.

14. **Long-Term Planning:** In cases of progressive kidney disease, healthcare providers assist patients in planning for the long term, including discussions about end-of-life care preferences and palliative care options.

15. **Empowerment:** Ultimately, healthcare providers empower kidney patients to take an active role in managing their health. They encourage open communication, shared decision-making, and self-advocacy.

The role of healthcare providers in developing personalized treatment plans for kidney patients is multifaceted, focusing not only on medical aspects but also on the holistic well-being of the individual. Personalization ensures that treatment aligns with the patient's unique circumstances, goals, and values.

Strategies for managing side effects and treatment-related challenges

Certainly, here are some strategies for managing side effects and treatment-related challenges for kidney patients:

1. Open Communication: Keep the lines of communication with your medical team open and honest.. Share any side effects or challenges you encounter during treatment promptly.

2. -Medication Adherence: Follow your prescribed medication regimen meticulously. Set up reminders if needed and discuss any concerns about

side effects with your healthcare provider.

3. Dietary Modifications: Follow your recommended diet plan, which may include restrictions on sodium, potassium, and phosphorus. Work with a registered dietitian to create enjoyable, kidney-friendly meals.

4. Fluid Management: If you have fluid restrictions, monitor your fluid intake carefully. Use small containers to track how much you drink throughout the day.

5. Exercise Regularly: Engage in physical activity suitable for your condition. Consult with your healthcare team to develop a safe and effective exercise routine.

6. Symptom Management: If you experience symptoms such as fatigue or pain, discuss them with your healthcare provider. They can suggest treatments or lifestyle adjustments to alleviate discomfort.

7. Stress Reduction: Practice stress-reduction techniques like meditation, deep breathing, or mindfulness to manage the emotional challenges of kidney disease and treatment.

8. Support Network: Build a support network of friends and family who understand your condition and can provide emotional support.

9. Support Groups: Join kidney disease support groups or online communities to connect with others facing similar challenges. Sharing experiences can provide valuable insights and emotional relief.

10. Regular Check-Ups: Attend all scheduled follow-up appointments to monitor your condition and make necessary adjustments to your treatment plan.

11. Stay Informed: Continuously educate yourself about kidney disease and its treatment

options. Knowledge empowers you to make informed decisions and advocate for your health.

12. Medication Management: If you experience side effects from medications, don't hesitate to discuss them with your healthcare provider. They can adjust your medication or suggest alternatives.

13. Emotional Well-Being: Prioritize your mental health. Seek professional support if you're dealing with anxiety, depression, or other emotional challenges.

14. Balance Activity and Rest: Find a balance between staying active and allowing your body to rest when needed. Listen to your body's signals and adjust your activities accordingly.

15. Financial Planning: Consider the financial aspects of treatment, including insurance coverage and potential costs. Discuss financial

concerns with your healthcare team or a financial counselor.

Chapter 4: Lifestyle and Diet for Kidney Health

Here are the thorough and interesting article that ably demonstrates the significant relationship between diet and lifestyle in your quest for kidney health:

The harmony of lifestyle and diet is demonstrated in the book The Symphony of Kidney Health.

The elaborate ballet of lifestyle and diet, a symphony in motion, with your kidneys as the star players, unfolds before you in the huge stage that is your body. We will take center stage in this chapter, shedding light on the significant relationship between your daily decisions and the colorful tapestry of renal health.

Act I: Lifestyle - The Dance of Decisions

This act will examine how your way of life choreographs the ballet's moves, with each decision a delicate pirouette or a powerful leap:

Daily choreography Daily habits govern your life, from the awakening at dawn to the sleep at dusk. Every decision you make, whether it's getting up early for a morning walk or easing into the day with stress-reduction measures, is a movement in your ballet that affects how well your kidneys function.

Stress is the shadow that hangs over your stage, posing a threat to tamp down the brilliance of your ballet. But don't worry, you have brushes nearby to sweep it away. Your tools are calm, exercise, and mindfulness; with each stroke, you are released from the burden of tension, allowing your kidneys to glow.

The same way a dancer seeks equilibrium in movement, you must do the same in life. When you achieve a harmonic balance between activity and rest, between work and recreation, your lifestyle will flourish. Your performance is made more complex and richer by the collective of your social relationships.

Act II: Diet – The Palette of Nutrition Artistry

Imagine your diet now as a colorful color palette, with each food serving as a pigment to paint your dietary canvas:

The nutritional spectrum is a rich tapestry made from the natural products that make up your food. The vibrant greens of leafy vegetables, the deep reds of antioxidant-rich berries, and the golden grains of healthy carbohydrates are all on your palate. Together, these colours form a culinary masterpiece that feeds your kidneys.

Water intake is the understated wash that creates the scene, or "brushstrokes of hydration." Your diet is the canvas on which your nutritional masterpiece is painted. The precise proportions of water brush strokes guarantee the purity and sparkle of your canvas.

There are shadows to be aware of among the vibrant colors and contrast. Dietary restrictions, such as those on salt, potassium, phosphorus, and protein, are frequently necessary for kidney function. Consider these limitations as subtle shading for balance and depth in your dietary artwork.

The Grand Finale: A Work of Art in Wellness

When the show is over, you will be in front of a wellness canvas that has been painted with the brushstrokes of your decisions and the vivid hues of your food. Dear reader, you are the choreographer of the ballet of your life, and the principal actors are your kidneys. Every day offers a fresh chance to mold this ballet and produce a masterpiece that depicts your journey toward robust, life-affirming kidney health.

Keep in mind that you are the conductor, leading the symphony of lifestyle and diet in the big stage of your live. They dance in perfect harmony as a celebration of the kidneys' vitality in this amazing performance we call life.

The significance of diet and lifestyle choices in kidney disease management.

Unveiling the Power of Diet and Lifestyle: Management Strategies for Kidney Disease

Consider your body as a highly tuned instrument, with nutrition and lifestyle as the keys that create the melodies of managing renal disease. The profound significance of these decisions in directing your path toward kidney health will be thoroughly discussed in this chapter.

Section 1: The Harmony of Nutrition

Diet supplies the energy needed by your body's complex machinery, including your kidneys. Your kidney function is strongly influenced by what you eat. We'll discuss the significance of:

- Balanced Nutrition: A harmonious combination of fresh fruits, vegetables, lean proteins, and whole grains is the foundation of a balanced diet, which is where the symphony starts.

Portion control helps you strike the correct balance between satisfying your body's nutritional needs and avoiding undue stress on your kidneys.

- Nutrient Prowess: Learn about the functions of particular nutrients, such as salt, potassium, and phosphorus, and how eating them in moderation helps your diet to be overall harmonious.

Section 2: The Conductor's Lifestyle

Taking Charge of Your Well-Being Your lifestyle decisions serve as the conductor's baton, guiding the group of everyday rituals you engage in. They have a significant impact on the health of your kidneys. We'll look at:

- Stress management: Stress is a common part of life's tempo. Utilize strategies like mindfulness, physical activity, and relaxation to manage your stress reaction and save your kidneys.

- Activity and Rest: Balance is essential, just as rhythm in music. Find the balance between exercise and rest that best promotes your wellbeing.

- Social Harmony: Just as a symphony uses a variety of instruments, forming social ties gives your life richness and significance. To improve your general quality of life, cultivate your relationships.

Section 3: The Interplay and Result

You'll start to see the results - the musical performance of renal disease management - as you investigate the harmonious interaction between nutrition and lifestyle:

- Symptom Management: By managing symptoms like fatigue, pain, and fluid imbalances, these harmonies can improve your general quality of life.

- Disease advancement: You can prevent kidney function loss by modifying your food and lifestyle to limit the advancement of renal disease.

- Empowerment: Acknowledging the significance of these decisions gives you the power to take an active role in maintaining the health of your kidneys and to navigate your journey with assurance and knowledge.

Section 4: Knowledge and Assistance

"Looking for the Maestros" The same way that a symphony depends on skilled musicians, your journey is aided by knowledge and assistance:

- Healthcare Professionals: Your maestros on this musical journey are nephrologists, dietitians, and therapists who will guide your decisions and arm you with the information you need.

- Support Groups and Online Communities: Interact with people in the same auditorium while exchanging notes and experiences.

You take on the role of a conductor, directing the symphony of your kidney disease management by realizing the profound significance of your diet and lifestyle decisions. You'll craft a path to kidney health that resonates with harmony, vitality, and empowerment as you fine-tune your diet and lifestyle.

Practical dietary guidelines and meal planning for kidney-friendly nutrition.

According to the Centers for Disease Control and Prevention (CDC), more than one in seven American persons have chronic kidney disease (CKD), although the majority don't become aware of their sickness until it is well along.

Even if you haven't been given a CKD diagnosis, it's a good idea to maintain your kidney health because late-stage kidney disease can lead to a buildup of waste in your body and a number of other health concerns, such as gout, bone disease, and heart disease.

One of the most critical things you can do to avoid or treat CKD is to keep a balanced diet. What you need to know about eating to maintain kidney health is covered here.

A kidney-friendly diet should restrict sodium, cholesterol, and fat, and instead focus on fruits, vegetables, whole grains, low-fat dairy, and lean meats (seafood, poultry, eggs, legumes, nuts, seeds, and soy products), explains Maruschak. People who have already been diagnosed with CKD may also need to limit some other minerals, she says.

Here are some methods to update your diet to maintain kidney function.

1. Portion Your Plate

As a general rule of thumb, Maruschak advocates using the MyPlate technique at every meal: Fill nearly half of your plate with vegetables and fruits, one-quarter with lean protein, and one-quarter with nutritious grains.

2. Limit Your Salt Intake

Sodium creeps its way into all sorts of places you wouldn't expect, especially packaged meals such as soups and breads. Limiting your sodium consumption helps keep your blood pressure under control. Aim for 2,300 milligrams per day — that's roughly 1 teaspoon of table salt — according to the Dietary Guidelines for Americans, 2020–2025, published by the U.S. Department of Agriculture (USDA).

If you're at risk of or already have high blood pressure, Maruschak advocates adopting a low-sodium diet, and specifically the Dietary Approaches to Stop Hypertension (DASH) eating plan. Also try these ways to keep your salt in check:

- **Limit ordering takeaway and eating at restaurants.** "Your food is frequently salted, and equipment used in restaurant kitchens may have sodium added, says Maruschak. Do some research before dining out. . You may occasionally find the sodium amount of dishes on the restaurant's website, she adds.

- **Cook at home with whole**, unprocessed foods. When you create meals at home with fresh ingredients, you control exactly how much sodium (and fat) goes into each bite.

- **Get creative with seasonings.** Maruschak advocates avoiding salt when cooking or at the meal. Instead, use spices, herbs, lemon, and other sodium-free ingredients.

- **Check the package.** Any prepared food with 20 percent or more of your daily requirement of salt is considered high-sodium. Choose soups, frozen meals, and other packaged items labeled as reduced or low-sodium or salt-free wherever you can.
- **Rinse canned items before eating**. This helps remove excess salt.

3. Watch Your Protein Intake

When you consume protein, your body creates waste that your kidneys filter. Although a balanced diet should contain enough amounts of protein, eating too much protein might strain your kidneys. A study from 2020 noted that while studies on the impact of a high-protein diet on general renal health is still developing, if you currently have CKD, your doctor will probably advise a lower-protein diet. When you consume too much protein, waste may accumulate in your blood and become difficult for your kidneys to filter out.

In order to slow the course of renal disease, Maruschak advises people with any stage of CKD who aren't receiving dialysis to keep their protein consumption between 0.6 and 0.8 grams per kilogram of body weight. According to the National Kidney Foundation of Hawaii, a person weighing 150 pounds (68 kg) would require 40 to 54 grams of protein per day, or about 4 to 6 ounces of protein derived from either plant or animal sources.. Make sure to consult a certified nutritionist to find out how much protein is ideal for you.

Whether or not you have CKD, choosing healthy protein sources and paying attention to your portion levels might be beneficial. Among the top protein sources are:

1. Lean meat, fish, or skinless poultry (one serving is about the size of a deck of cards, weighing between two and three ounces)
2. Eggs
3. Dairy (one amount of yogurt, milk, or cheese equals one ounce,

or around the size of your two thumbs put together),
4. Beans, chickpeas, lentils, and peas (a serving is equal to 1/2 cup)
5. Nuts (1/4 cup is one portion)

Tips for staying active and maintaining a healthy lifestyle

Tips for Maintaining an Active and Vibrant Lifestyle: Sculpting a Healthy Lifestyle
Staying active and adopting a healthy lifestyle are the colorful strokes that illuminate your canvas in the magnificent work of art that is life. Here, we'll provide you with some useful advice so that you can traverse the course of kidney illness with vigor, strength, and wellbeing.
1. Find Activities You Love: Opt for pursuits that make you happy. No matter what you enjoy doing—dancing, hiking, swimming, or practicing yoga—staying active becomes a pleasure rather than a job.
2. Establish realistic objectives Set reasonable fitness objectives that take into account your

present health and fitness level. As your strength and endurance grow, gradually up the intensity and duration of your workouts.

3. Establish a Routine: Create a regular workout schedule that combines flexibility, strength training, and a variety of cardiovascular exercises. The secret to enjoying the advantages of an active lifestyle is consistency.

4. Involve a Friend: Tell a friend or family member about your fitness journey. Together, you can increase motivation and enjoy your workout more.

5. Pay Attention to Your Body: Keep a watchful eye on your body's reaction to exercise. Consult a medical professional if you develop pain, discomfort, or unusual exhaustion. You can modify your routine with their assistance to fit your demands.

Keep Hydrated: **6. For the health of your kidneys in particular, proper hydration is crucial. To keep the proper fluid balance when exercising, drink water before, during, and after.

Warm-up and cool-down exercises: Always warm up your

muscles before exercising, and cool down afterward to avoid muscular soreness and lower your chance of injury.

Integrate strength training: **8. Strengthening and preserving your muscles is essential. To support general fitness, incorporate resistance workouts into your program, such as lifting weights or utilizing resistance bands.

9. Mindful Movement: Mind-body exercises such as yoga and tai chi not only increase flexibility and balance but also relax the body and mind and lower stress levels, which is good for kidney health.

10. Seek Professional Guidance: Speak with a physical therapist or fitness trainer, particularly if you have certain health issues or restrictions. They can create an exercise plan specifically for you.

11. Give sleep first priority: A good night's sleep is crucial for recuperation and general health. To complement your busy lifestyle, aim for 7-8 hours of good sleep each night.

12. Healthy Eating: Add a balanced diet to your active lifestyle. Choose kidney-friendly foods, with a focus on fresh produce, lean meats, and whole grains. To receive individualized nutrition advice, speak with a licensed dietitian.

13. Control your stress: Include stress-reduction practices like mindfulness, meditation, or deep breathing in your daily routine. Stress reduction has a favorable effect on kidney health.

14. Stay Informed: Continue your education regarding renal illness and how to treat it. You can make wise decisions regarding your lifestyle and health when you are well-informed.

Keep in mind that your path to living a healthy lifestyle is individual to you. These pointers will serve as your waypoints as you travel the road to continuing to be active and vibrant. Accept every day as a chance to improve your health and create a masterpiece of vitality.

Chapter 5: Overcoming Obstacles and Managing the Storms of Kidney Disease

Storms are a part of the journey with renal illness, but so is resiliency. With tactics for managing symptoms, guidance for navigating mental storms, and encouraging true-life accounts of people who have not just weathered but triumphed over these problems, Chapter 5 is your harbor during choppy waters.

Strategies for Managing Symptoms, Pain, and Fatigue in

The Compass for Symptom Management Fatigue, pain, and discomfort are symptoms that come and go like erratic currents. Here, we provide a trustworthy compass to guide them:
- Understanding Symptoms: Your compass is knowledge. Discover the signs and symptoms

of kidney illness, their likely causes, and how to tell them apart.

-Medication Management: You may use drugs as part of your treatment plan to control symptoms. We walk you through your drug alternatives and any possible adverse effects.

- Pain Management Techniques: Learn about a variety of pain-relieving strategies, including prescription drugs, physical therapy, and complementary treatments like acupuncture.

- Combating Fatigue: When fatigue strikes, it might seem like a never-ending tempest. Learn useful methods for preserving energy and regaining vitality.

Advice on dealing with stress, anxiety, and depression related to kidney disease

The Compassion for Emotional Well-Being (TCEB) Like the tides of the sea, emotions can ebb and flow. Using the advice in this section, you can weather emotional storms:

- How to Deal with Stress: Stress is like rough seas. To find peace in the midst of the storm, practice stress-reduction methods like mindfulness, meditation, and deep breathing.

Anxiety and kidney disease Anxiety may accompany you on this trip. Learn how kidney disease can cause anxiety as well as coping mechanisms.

-Overcoming Depression: Although depression is a heavy cloud, there is still hope. Learn coping strategies, therapeutic alternatives, and the value of asking for help.

Real-life stories of individuals who have overcome challenges.

Real-life stories are your way's lighthouses, according to the "Beacons of Resilience" program. Meet people who have confronted renal disease head-on:
- Stories of Triumph: These people have not only endured, but also flourished, demonstrating the tenacity of the human spirit.

- Lessons Learned: Gain knowledge from their experiences, such as the difficulties they overcame and the tactics they used to succeed.

- Community and Support: These tales highlight the value of having a network of friends and family who can lean on when times are tough.

<u>Look into these real life stories</u>
Conclusion:

Your road map for overcoming the psychological and physical difficulties of renal disease is Chapter 5. You are prepared to navigate your ship over even the roughest seas with the aid of information, a toolbox of tactics, and the motivation of true stories. Although the storms may rage, you have what it takes to endure them, find moments of peace amid the mayhem, and come out on the other side stronger, wiser, and more forgiving than before.

Chapter 6: Empowering Your Mindset:

As you traverse the difficulties of renal disease, Chapter 6 is your doorway to transformation—a manual that enables you to shape your mindset into a fortress of resilience, positivism, and steadfast determination.

The Power of Positive Thinking in managing Kidney Disease

The Science of Positive Thinking
- Examine the scientific evidence supporting the remarkable influence of positive thinking on your general health and well-being.
- Explore the research showing how optimism can strengthen your immune system, reduce stress, and improve your quality of life.

1.2 Cultivating Optimism- Arm yourself with useful methods for fostering optimism, such as gratitude exercises, daily affirmations, and visualization techniques.

- Accept these strategies as the seeds of optimism that will grow in your day-to-day experiences and shift your viewpoint to the more positive aspects of life.

1.3 Combating Unfavorable Thoughts

- Face and vanquish any negative shadows that may stand in your way.

- Acquire techniques for challenging and swapping out self-defeating beliefs for empowering ones, turning roadblocks into stepping stones.

Strengthening Resilience

Explore the idea of resilience, the cornerstone of your capacity to overcome hardship, in this section.

- Recognize how your resilience will help you navigate renal disease's storms.

2.2 Strategies for Increasing Resilience

- Equip yourself with a wide range of resilience-enhancing strategies. These methods strengthen your inner fortitude by enhancing your problem-solving abilities and emotional control.

- Recognize the value of asking for help and accept that doing so is a sign of strength rather than a sign of weakness.

2.3 Stories of Resilience - Find motivation from real-life examples of people who overcame hardships caused by renal illness to not only survive but also thrive.

- Through this stories, learn how resilience has the potential to transform, and use that knowledge to inspire your self

Meditation and Mindfulness

3.1 The Mindfulness Art

- Master the practice of mindfulness, which can help you stay in the present moment, reduce stress, and promote general well-being.

- Recognize the significant advantages of mindfulness in coping with the emotional turbulence of kidney disease.

3.2 Mindfulness Practices for Kidney Health

- Examine specialized meditation techniques created to promote kidney health. These techniques emphasize emotional stability, pain control, and relaxation.
- Accept meditation as your dependable ally on the road to complete kidney wellness.

Adopting a Warrior Mindset

A Warrior's Viewpoint
- Learn from those who have adopted this approach in their fight against kidney disease to put yourself in the mindset of a warrior. - Learn about their bravery, tenacity, and unflinching resilience in their stories.
Building mental toughness
- Arm yourself with methods for developing mental toughness, such as goal-setting, self-control, and flexibility.
- Unleash the warrior within to face adversity head-on and be prepared to overcome any obstacle life may throw your way.
Conclusion:

In Chapter 6, you are encouraged to design your own thinking and build an impregnable fortress that endures renal disease's challenges. By strengthening your thinking, you'll travel this path not as a victim of events but rather as a tough, upbeat, and unyielding warrior, destined for success and happiness.

You will discover your enormous potential as you go through Chapter 6's scenery, a potential to cultivate a mindset that will be your greatest ally as you travel through kidney disease and beyond. This mentality is one of resiliency, optimism, and steadfast resolve, prepared to turn problems into victories, setbacks into stepping stones, and hurdles into chances.

Keep in mind that your thinking serves as your compass as you navigate the maze of life. It shines a light of hope even in the most difficult circumstances. As you develop and strengthen your thinking, you take control of your own future and are better equipped to face kidney illness head-on and come out on the other side stronger, wiser, and ready for a life of limitless potential.

You get a little bit closer to understanding the enormous power you have within you with each page of this chapter that you flip. Your mindset is the foundation of your path, so by strengthening it, you give yourself the capacity to accept the difficulties and successes that lie ahead, to thrive, and to flourish in the face of renal illness and everything else.

Chapter 7: Navigating Treatment Options:

Introduction:
Your guide through the maze of kidney disease therapy options is Chapter 7. Here, we look at the several options you have, from drugs to dialysis and transplantation, to assist you in making decisions about your road to kidney wellness.

Treatments and Medication

1.1 Kidney Disease Medicines

Explore the universe of drugs used to treat renal illness, including ACE inhibitors and diuretics.

- Recognize how these medications function, any possible adverse effects, and how they affect the progression of the condition.

1.2 Anemia Management - Learn about the management of anemia, which is frequently accompanied with kidney disease. Learn about iron supplements and erythropoietin-stimulating agents (ESAs).

- Learn how managing your anemia can enhance your overall quality of life and energy levels.

Dialysis is your lifeline

2.1 Peritoneal and hemodialysis

- Examine hemodialysis and peritoneal dialysis, the two main forms of dialysis.

- Learn about each method's steps, advantages, drawbacks, and required lifestyle changes.

Options for Dialysis Access

- Examine the many hemodialysis access options available, such as arteriovenous fistulas, grafts, and catheters.

- Recognize the significance of maintaining and caring for vascular access.

The Transplantation Process

3.1 The Process of Transplant Evaluation

- Succeed in the challenging kidney transplant evaluation procedure, which includes matching and compatibility tests as well as medical and psychological evaluations.

- Find out the requirements that determine if you might make a good transplant candidate.

Finding a Reliable Donor

- Be aware of the challenges involved in obtaining a compatible kidney donor, including choices for live and deceased donors.

- Examine the logistical and emotional ramifications of the donor selection procedure.

Life After Transplantation

4.1 The Experience of Transplant Surgery

- Get ready for the transplant surgical procedure, including the preoperative steps and the following recovery period.
- Learn what to anticipate at this important stage of your renal wellness journey.

4.2 Post-Transplant Maintenance and Care

- Get familiar with the crucial post-transplant treatment schedule, which includes immunosuppressant medication, monitoring, and follow-up consultations.
- Learn how to prolong the life and preserve the health of your transplanted kidney.

Conclusion:

You gain a thorough awareness of kidney disease treatment options in Chapter 7, which will help you make decisions about your route to kidney wellness. Always keep in mind that each decision you make will bring you one step closer to a healthier, more fulfilling life as you travel the routes of drugs, dialysis, and transplantation. With the knowledge and assurance to manage your renal health and embrace the prospects of the future, your journey continues.

Chapter 8: Empowering Your Support Network:

Introduction:
Chapter 8 offers advice on how to make the most of your network of friends and family while you face the difficulties of renal illness. Here, we discuss the value of friends, family, medical professionals, and support networks in building a solid foundation for your journey to renal wellness.

Family and friends serve as the foundation of support

The Family's Function

- Examine how important it is for families to help one another emotionally, practically, and morally.
- Recognize how your kidney illness journey can enhance family ties via transparent communication and shared responsibility.
Explore the special kind of assistance that friends provide, from being sympathetic listeners to offering company and encouragement.
- Acquire the skills to express your requirements to peers and build a network of people who can help you outside of your family.

Healthcare Providers as Partners

The Doctor-Patient Relationship in Nephrology
- Recognize your nephrologist's crucial position as your go-to authority on kidney disease.
- Understand how to ask questions, encourage effective communication, and actively engage in treatment decisions.

The Essential Function of Specialists

- Examine the contributions made by numerous experts, including nutritionists, social workers, and mental health specialists.

- Consider how their knowledge can improve your overall health and offer holistic care.

Online Communities and Support Groups

Support Groups Have Power

- Understand the importance of participating in live or online support groups for renal disease.

- Discover the value of shared knowledge, experiences, and emotional support as you travel.

Finding Your Way Around Online Communities

- Examine the advantages of interacting with online forums and communities dedicated to renal disease.

- Recognize the benefits of online communities, guidance, and platforms for sharing your experiences.

Advocacy and Self-Advocacy

Becoming a Supporter

- Learn how advocating for better resources and care can help you spread the word about kidney illness.

- Learn about chances to join groups that advocate for people with kidney illness.

Self-Advocacy Skills

- Work on your self-advocacy abilities so you can actively take part in healthcare decisions.

- Acquire knowledge about asking questions, getting second opinions, and managing your health.

Conclusion:

The transformational role of your support system in your experience with renal disease is highlighted in Chapter 8. You build a strong foundation that equips you to meet the challenges ahead by cultivating good relationships with family, friends, healthcare professionals, and support groups. Your support system serves as both a safety net to catch you in difficult times and a driving force to help you achieve kidney wellness. Remember that you are not alone as you begin this chapter; the courage and support of those who are at your side will enrich your trip.

Conclusion: Making Your Way to Kidney Wellness

We consider the amazing adventure you've been on via the pages of this book as we come to the end of this transforming voyage. Your journey to renal wellness has been characterized by wisdom, tenacity, and an unyielding commitment to not only survive kidney disease but to thrive in it.

Consider the chapters that have helped you navigate the complexity of renal illness as you reflect on your journey. You've learned a plethora of information and ideas about anything from the fundamentals of kidney function to mastering kidney-friendly nutrition, evaluating treatment options to empowering your mentality.

Accepting Resilience:

You have discovered the extraordinary power of resilience on your trip. You've mastered the art of adapting, overcoming hardship with bravery, and weathering life's storms to become stronger. Your path has served as a tribute to both your inner fortitude and the human spirit's resiliency.

The function of support is:

You've come to realize how important your support system—family, friends, medical professionals, and other warriors—has been to you during this journey. They have served as the pillars you have relied on and the motivation that has kept you motivated during trying times.

In the Future, There Are Many Possibilities:

Knowing that your route to renal wellness continues as you close out this chapter of your journey is comforting. You are prepared to welcome an uncertain future because you have knowledge, resilience, and a strong network of allies. You have the skills and the spirit to succeed whether you're managing your kidney health through dietary modifications, going through dialysis, or starting the life-changing adventure of a transplant.

A Note of Appreciation

We really appreciate you choosing to entrust us with your kidney wellness journey. We have had the privilege of serving as your tour guide, and we are motivated by your unrelenting dedication to good health.

Your Hope-Leaf Legacy

As you put this book away, keep in mind that your journey has served as a source of inspiration for others who are dealing with renal disease as well as a tale of personal victory. Your life lessons, tenacity, and tenacity serve as a beacon for those who travel a similar journey.

In conclusion:

Your path to renal health is a monument to the human spirit's capacity to thrive in the face of difficulty. May you begin the chapters that lie ahead with the unshakeable conviction that you have the power, the wisdom, and the resources to build a future rich in health, vigor, and limitless opportunity.

With sincere hopes for your ongoing health,

(Dr. Sharon C. Stallworth)

Appendix

Recommended Reads

With the help of these enlightening books, you may improve your knowledge of kidney disease, wellness practices, and personal development. Whether you're looking for inspiration, useful advice, or in-depth medical expertise, these books provide insightful information to enhance your experience.

1. J. Stewart Cameron's book "The Kidney Patient's Book: New Treatment, New Hope" An extensive handbook explaining lifestyle modifications, treatment alternatives, and renal disease. Kidney patients and their families can benefit greatly from the insights offered by Dr. Cameron.

2. Michelle L. Owens, MD, "The First Year: Hypertension" - This

book provides a patient-centered method for comprehending and controlling hypertension, a frequent side effect of kidney illness.

3. Lissa Rankin, MD's book "Mind Over Medicine: Scientific Proof That You Can Heal Yourself" Examine the fundamental healing relationship between the mind and body. The work of Dr. Rankin encourages a comprehensive approach to wellbeing.

4. L.S. Newton's book "The Transplant Journey: A Guide to Transplant: Extraordinary Stories, Hope, and Encouragement" This book offers helpful transplant advice and motivational transplant stories for anyone contemplating or recovering from a kidney transplant.

5. Susan Zogheib, "The Renal Diet Cookbook for Beginners: Your Complete Guide to Managing Kidney Disease" A useful cookbook that offers dietary recommendations and kidney-friendly dishes to maintain the health of your kidneys.

6. Barbara L. Trettin's book "Kidney Transplantation: A Guide to the Care of Kidney Transplant Recipients" Learn everything there is to know about kidney transplantation, from pre- through post-transplant care.

7. Eckhart Tolle, "The Power of Now: A Guide to Spiritual Enlightenment" This timeless spiritual manual provides guidance on practicing mindfulness, lowering stress levels, and living in the present.

8. Bob Roth's book "Strength in Stillness: The Power of Transcendental Meditation" Examine how meditation can help you feel better and reduce stress.

9. Shawn Achor's book "The Happiness Advantage: How a Positive Brain Fuels Success in Work and Life" Learn about the science of happiness and how adopting a positive outlook can enhance your life's overall quality.

10. Angela Duckworth's book "Grit: The Power of Passion and Perseverance" Examine the idea of grit and how perseverance and

tenacity are essential for conquering obstacles.

These suggested books present a variety of viewpoints on kidney health, growth as a person, and wellbeing. Whether you're looking for motivation or medical expertise, these books offer insightful information to help you on your path to a happier, healthier life.

Kidney Disease Resources Directory

Having trustworthy information, resources, and support is crucial on your path to renal wellness. The list of businesses, websites, and support groups that can offer kidney disease patients and their families vital support, direction, and a feeling of belonging is provided below.

NKF, the National Kidney Foundation

- https://www.kidney.org/On the website kidney.org

- A premier group devoted to kidney disease support, treatment, and prevention. On their website, you can get patient resources, instructional materials, and details about kidney health.

Kidney Patients' American Association (AAKP)

Online at [www.aakp.org]Link: https://www.aakp.org

- Kidney patients and their families can receive support, advocacy, and instructional materials from AAKP. Visit their website to learn about their patient-centered initiatives and educational publications.

Digestive and Kidney Diseases and Diabetes National Institute (NIDDK)

• [www.niddk.nih.gov] is the website.(www.niddk.nih.gov)

NIDDK, a division of the National Institutes of Health (NIH), provides up-to-date research information, treatment options, and extensive information on kidney health.

Network for Renal Support (RSN)

- https://www.rsnhope.org/A URL for https://www.rsnhope.org

- RSN is a patient-centered group that provides kidney disease patients with informational materials, advocacy, and support. They have information and motivational patient stories on their website.

Native Dialysis Patients (DPC)
[www.dialysispatients.org] is the website.The   website dialysispatients.org
- DPC supports the community of dialysis patients and offers helpful tools and resources, such as information on patient rights and legislative updates, for those receiving dialysis.

Living Transplant (UNOS)
[www.transplantliving.org] is the website.This   website, transplantliving.org,
This website provides extensive information   on   organ transplantation, including kidney transplantation,   eligibility requirements, and patient tales. United   Network   for   Organ Sharing (UNOS)is in charge of it.

MyFoodCoach   created   by Davita
-
[www.myfoodcoach.davita.com] is the website.via MyFoodCoach on Davita.com
- For those with renal disease, MyFoodCoach is a useful source for   meal   planning,   kidney-

friendly recipes, and nutritional advice.

Community Emergency Response Kidney (KCER)

[www.kcercoalition.com] is the website.the kcercoalition.com website

- KCER offers resources and information on emergency preparedness that are specifically designed to meet the requirements of renal patients.

Information about COVID-19 and Kidney Disease

The CDC, or the Centers for Disease Control and Prevention,(https://www.cdc.gov/coronavirus/2019-ncov/healthy-individuals/need-extra-precautions.html)

Resources for the National Kidney Foundation's COVID-19(Source: https://www.kidney.org/coronavirus/covid-19-kidney-disease)